A Crash Course

on

Prostate Cancer

A Crash Course

on

Prostate Cancer

From

One *Woman's* Perspective

Lynne Rosenberg

iUniverse, Inc.

New York Lincoln Shanghai

A Crash Course on Prostate Cancer
From One Woman's Perspective

iUniverse books may be ordered through booksellers or by contacting:

iUniverse
2021 Pine Lake Road, Suite 100
Lincoln, NE 68512
www.iuniverse.com
1-800-Authors (1-800-288-4677)

ISBN-13: 978-0-595-39823-2 (pbk)
ISBN-13: 978-0-595-84229-2 (ebk)
ISBN-10: 0-595-39823-5 (pbk)
ISBN-10: 0-595-84229-1 (ebk)

Printed in the United States of America

Contents

Introduction

It was two years ago when I first realized that I knew nothing about prostate cancer. Prostate cancer is not an easy topic to just start talking about and not a topic that usually captures people's attention. That is, unless of course you love someone who is facing prostate cancer.

There are several important points that women need to hear and understand as they move through those days surrounding this possibility...the possibility that the man they love may have prostate cancer. And of course, this is the worst possible time to be able to concentrate and remember those vital pieces of information.

That is why this book is written by me—a woman who has been there. A woman who wanted and needed to speak with another woman who had lived through this. But doctors were hesitant to suggest someone to speak with because "everyone's experience is different." This is true; however there are some emotions and fears that we all face during this time. And that is where this book comes in.

This book is intended as a crash course on prostate cancer from a woman's perspective.

The End of the Story First

For people such as my sister, who always sneak a peek at the end of the book, I have decided to wrap things up in the very beginning. The purpose behind this decision is very simple. It is my goal to have women understand the previously unknown territory of a man's prostate and his risk for prostate cancer. It is my goal to have women be a part of the solution in identifying prostate cancer in its early stages. And for that reason, I am providing essential, bare-bone facts up front.

There are two essential screening tests for prostate cancer:

- The first is the Prostate-specific antigen (PSA) blood test. Simply stated, this is a test that examines a protein in the blood—the prostate specific antigen. The level of PSA rises in men who may have an enlarged prostate, an infection of the prostate gland or cancer of the prostate. (www.dva.gov.au/media/publicat/2001/prostate/glos-sary.htm.)

  - This blood test needs to be done each year if the man in your life is at least 45 years of age or older, has a family history of prostate cancer, or is of African descent.

  - You need to obtain a copy of the results of his PSA blood test. Before you file it at home with your medical records you need to compare the newest PSA blood test result with previous results. You are looking for an increase in the PSA level over time referred to as the PSA velocity.

• The PSA blood test does not and cannot diagnosis prostate cancer. Only biopsies of the prostate gland can diagnosis cancer.

• The second test may be a difficult subject to discuss but a digital rectal exam performed by a competent physician provides important information by detecting changes in a man's prostate gland.

If necessary, a biopsy of the prostate is done to diagnosis prostate cancer. This biopsy may result in a bloody ejaculate preventing sexual intercourse for days or weeks.

And if there is a conclusive diagnosis of cancer, I suggest you read the rest of this book for a crash course on prostate cancer.

The Rest of the Story

HOW COME EVERYONE KNOWS SOMEONE?

Where do I begin? My husband has prostate cancer. When my husband Mark was diagnosed he was just 51 years old. I didn't know what to do. I searched the internet for medical information, support groups and references. I spent hours in neighborhood bookstores and bought every book I could find. I told everyone I came into contact with, from the dry cleaners to perfect strangers in a store that my husband had cancer. But I still felt lost. I needed to speak with other women who had gone through this with their husbands or partners.

There is very little research investigating a couple's response to prostate cancer, especially from the emotional or psychological viewpoint. What I have learned since that time was that my response was normal. Most people and most couples when confronted with prostate cancer scramble to learn everything they can about the prostate. They try to educate themselves about what a cancer diagnosis means in terms of stage of the disease, prognosis, potential treatments as well as consequences of treatment, essentially a "crash course" on prostate cancer.

What was most surprising to me during this time was that most people already knew someone with prostate cancer. Conversations usually entailed murmurs of sympathy and the stories of people they knew who had prostate cancer who were "just fine." I never found comfort in these words. Either the person they knew was older than my husband or their well intended words scared me even more. To be fair, prostate cancer and prostate cancer screenings run in cycles as a news topic and in health fairs. But what if the reality is different? What if more men are being diagnosed and diagnosed at a younger age? What impact does this have on their lives? When a man is older (seventy or so) when he is diagnosed with prostate cancer, the common theory is that he will die from something other than prostate cancer. But, when a man is like my husband, and diagnosed at a younger age, the cancer may be more aggressive and require more aggressive surveillance and management. How many middle-aged women are finding their lives "turned upside down" by the possibility of prostate cancer? And how do they cope with the implications of such a diagnosis?

I remember many people telling me, "This is not happening to you. Be strong". But of course it was happening to me. My life was changing and I had no control over the situation. And I was scared. I was scared because of everything I didn't know and everything I feared I would lose. Little is known about a couple's response and adaptation to a cancer diagnosis but it is acknowledged that prostate cancer in particular affects the couple, not just the patient.

Prostate cancer is unusual in that it is still cancer but also has a direct impact on a man's sexuality and urinary continence. How do you provide support to the most significant person in your life when you have no idea of the threat they are facing.

What does prostate cancer mean to a man? Is cancer foremost in his mind? Or is he more concerned with the surgery and the possible consequences of the surgery. What does it mean to a man in his fifties if he suddenly cannot have an erection? If I were a man, and a husband what would it mean to me? I kept thinking of an episode of Seinfeld. Seinfeld for those of you not familiar with the show was a very successful sitcom about "nothing". Each episode focused on the lives of four friends: Jerry, Elaine, Kramer and George. In one of the episodes Elaine was talking about her personal experiences with a new boyfriend. In speaking with Jerry she said she couldn't fully understand a man's sexuality because she didn't have "access to the equipment 24 hours a day." That is the way I felt. How was I supposed to cope with my husband's diagnosis of prostate cancer, surgery and other unknowns when I didn't know what it meant for him? Since that time, I have learned through first hand experience what prostate cancer means to a man, a woman and a couple. I have kept informed of relevant research studies focusing on how prostate cancer and its treatment affect a man and listed them in the selected readings section.

This book does not have all of the answers. No single book or resource can provide that. It is not intended to be a medical book. It is deliberately intended to be a heart to heart crash course on prostate cancer for women. It is hoped that this book can help balance those thoughts you may be having and let you know you are not alone, your thoughts are not irrational and you are indeed going through this experience. It is true that every single man that experiences prostate cancer will have his own unique story. And, it is also true that if there is a woman standing beside him, she will have her own perception of those same events.

This book is intended specifically for the woman who is walking beside the man, the woman who is the unexpected participant in his prostate journey.

SO WHY SHOULD YOU READ THIS BOOK?

You need to read this book to get all of the information you can, from all of the relevant sources you can. The fact that my husband and I are both health professionals gave us a unique view into our world that left us baffled at the gaps in care, information and resources. Being a physician, Mark had an advantage that most men do not have. He was able to order his own lab studies. He had access to other physicians and could state his reasons for requesting more diagnostic studies. The PSA blood test will be discussed in the next section but for now, it is important to know that Mark's PSA was always within normal limits. Every physician Mark worked with and spoke with felt there was no need for alarm. The blood test was normal and besides….Mark looked and felt great.

A very important reason to read this book is because you need to understand that most of the health care professionals you encounter will have no first hand experience of prostate cancer. A male urologist may understand the surgical procedure and the latest recommended treatment, but unless he has actually had a prostate biopsy and cancer diagnosis, he would have no idea what you are experiencing. The nurses in the office may be primarily women and also cannot usually speak from first hand experience. We were just one of the many patients and their families in the crowded waiting room isolated in their own world of worry. Of course, this is true for most medical diagnoses but in this situation women can help make the difference for the men in their lives.

Through this experience it became clear that men, who have experienced prostate cancer and its aftermath, do not have candid discussions with their doctors. Call it male bravado but discussing rectal exams, impotence and incontinence is off limits for many men. Perhaps the medical profession needs to think twice about the time they spend with these patients. The people in these situations, both physicians and patients, need to understand they are part of the solution for other men yet to come. The more information these men provide, the more candid they can be, the better the medical community can refine screening for prostate cancer and provide the necessary support for those men and their families facing cancer and its effect on their lives.

HOW OUR PROSTATE JOURNEY BEGAN

Each man who is faced with a rising PSA and his partner will have a unique experience for obvious reasons. Each one of us handles stress differently; each one of us has different support strategies. And each of our relationships is different.

Our relationship and our family have revolved around the practice of emergency medicine for over 25 years. Mark is a physician who works in an Emergency Department and I am a Registered Nurse.

Mark is the guy next door who is riding his bike, going to the gym, taking his vitamins and scheduling annual physicals. He has boundless energy and truly enjoys every waking moment. He is up at 4 a.m., goes to the gym and arrives at the Emergency Department by 7 a.m. for a 12 hour shift of seeing patients. I get exhausted just thinking about it! If you could see Mark, you would consider him the picture of health.

Our prostate journey began as an unexpected diversion in our lives. One day we just followed the normal routine and the next day Mark decided to follow his gut instinct. Mark had a nagging feeling about his latest PSA. Although the test was still normal and our family doctor said his exam was normal, Mark was not reassured. So he asked a colleague, who was also an urologist, to do an ultrasound. Mark's suspicions proved correct. The ultrasound showed a mass in his prostate gland. We didn't know it at the time, but life as we knew it had just ended.

Our urologist told us that prostate cancer would bring us closer together. That is quite an interesting comment which I have thought about many times throughout the past year. Having the benefit of hindsight I can say that our whole relationship has been redefined. However, I also think a relationship is constantly changing, especially a long-term relationship so cancer is just one more unexpected event. Are we closer? It depends on which day you ask me!

The Nuts and Bolts

I admit that statistics and textbook type information can be boring and monotonous. But in this case, I think it is essential to understand the basics of prostate cancer. Who is the typical guy walking around with prostate cancer? What are the screening tests? How is a diagnosis made? What is a biopsy of the prostate? Trust me, I am not writing a medical school book but rather giving you some "cliff notes" which just might come in handy. And I think it is important to become familiar with some of the medical "jargon" associated with prostate cancer so you can be an active participant in the decisions to be made.

PROSTATE CANCER STATISTICS

This little book would not be complete without some basic information regarding the prostate, the PSA blood test and prostate cancer. There are many excellent resources on the market today that can give you as much information as you want or need. Dr. Patrick Walsh's book, *Guide to Surviving Prostate Cancer*, was the most comprehensive book for us and also served as a reference throughout those first few months of confusion. I still refer back to it even today. However, there are also many excellent resources on the internet, the American Cancer Society and the American Foundation for Urologic Disease, Inc. to name a few.

I have used the American Cancer Society (ACS) as a reference for providing prostate cancer statistics. There is some discrepancy in the literature as to how data is collected, how cases are estimated and trended as well as reporting procedures. Regardless of the source, however, the main message is clear: ***Prostate cancer is a leading cause of cancer death in American men.***

It is estimated that during the year 2006, approximately 234,460 men will be diagnosed with prostate cancer in the United States (ACS, 2006). The good news is that more men are being diagnosed with prostate cancer primarily due to the PSA blood test as a screening tool. Earlier detection improves survival rates as the cancer may be found at an earlier stage. The ACS reports that modern detection methods and treatments have led to an annual drop in death rate of approximately 3.5 percent.

The ACS offers statistics per age category that are of interest in prostate cancer. For men between the ages of 40 to 59, *one (1) man out of every 44 men* may develop prostate cancer. This rate increases to *one (1) out of every seven (7)* men in the 60 to 79 years of age category. More than 70% of all prostate cancer cases are diagnosed in men older than 65 years of age.

Other established risk factors for prostate cancer are ethnicity and family history of the disease. African American men and Jamaican men of African descent have the highest prostate cancer incidence rates in the world (Cancer Facts & Figures,

2004). And a family predisposition for prostate cancer or family history accounts for 5-10% of all cases.

Why should these statistics be important to you?

Because many times, there are no symptoms associated with prostate cancer. This is especially true in the early stages. This is the best time for screening and for being proactive. At this time, there are no medical or scientific organizations that advocate *routine* testing for the early detection of prostate cancer. It is recommended that healthcare professionals discuss the *option* of a PSA blood test and digital rectal exam with their patients, allowing men to make individualized decisions about testing. The ACS recommends that health care professionals *offer* these screening tests to their male patients beginning at the age of 50 and at age 45 for those men who are at high risk.

WHAT IS THE PSA?

Prostate-specific antigen (PSA) is a protein produced by the cells of the prostate gland. PSA levels have been used as a cancer screening tool since approved by the Federal Drug Administration (FDA) in 1986. This antigen is measured by a simple blood test. The lab's "normal range" is 0–4.0 and the results are usually reported in ng/ml or nanograms per milliliter. (A nanogram is one-billionth of a gram and a milliliter is one-thousandth of a liter.) This range of 0–4.0 ng/ml is used as a cutoff point to separate men who are less likely to have prostate cancer from those for whom further testing may be needed. Even if the result falls within the normal range the doctor may decide that further testing may be needed. And if the result is above the "normal range" it does not necessarily mean prostate cancer but should be discussed with your doctor to decide if there is a need for further testing.

You may remember that I said my husband's PSA was always normal. Mark's PSA results never rose beyond 3.16 ng/ml. The results of his annual PSA tests were rising over the years but still considered normal. This increase is called the PSA velocity. The ACS notes that if the PSA increases more than 0.75 ng/ml over an 18 month period cancer may be present and a biopsy should be considered. Studies by Freedland (2005) report, "…clearly limitations to the PSA test exist, it still remains the best prostate cancer marker for detection and prognostication available to date, particularly when coupled with looking at changes in the PSA level with time."

Recent studies have shown that perhaps the upper range of normal for a PSA needs to be lowered to 2.5 ng/ml. Dr. Ian Thompson (2004) states that "the medical community and the general public need to get away from the concept that the PSA is either positive or negative and that biopsies should be performed automatically in response to a certain PSA value." Dr. Thompson recommends that "all factors, age, ethnicity, family history and the results of the rectal examination, be considered along with the PSA level when trying to decide whether to proceed to biopsy."

Why should this interest you?

Because you are probably the one who handles your family's medical records. The doctor's office of today may include multiple practitioners, double bookings, changes in office staff and a hectic pace. If you have insurance, your provider or coverage may change. That is why you need to keep a copy of your families' health care records in your own home. And you need to compare those records year to year. It is significant because you may be the one to detect any change in PSA lab results. It is important to remember that the PSA blood test does not and cannot diagnose prostate cancer. It is only a screening tool and a monitoring tool. An actual biopsy of the prostate is needed to determine the presence of cancer.

THE RECTAL EXAM—A TOUCHY TOPIC

Another "touchy" topic is the rectal exam. Part of Mark's annual physical was a rectal exam by our family doctor. However, when Mark had a rectal exam by the urologist, he said he had never had quite such an exam! It may have been uncomfortable, but that rectal exam detected the mass in Mark's prostate before the ultrasound. So let me ask you this. As a woman, we go to the gynecologist every year (or at least we should), lay with our legs in stirrups and submit to internal exams and Pap smears. Why shouldn't the men in our lives go to the urologist office and get an annual rectal exam and PSA? It has been said that a rectal exam is only as good as the practitioner doing it. Some of the true experts are urologists and if the man in your life is at risk for prostate cancer, he deserves the very best in surveillance testing. And that my friend may be an annual check up with an urologist.

You may find yourself in the position of talking to your partner about the need for further testing. The man in your life is sitting across from you at the kitchen table and you want him to do what! Get a rectal exam? Have a blood test? You're kidding! Actually, you've never been more serious in your life. And if you are a woman like me, you know how to nag and cajole to get your point across. All you are asking for is a simple examination each year to detect a potentially lethal change that can affect both of you. And being the woman in the house, you will probably be the one to bring up the subject or even make the appointment.

Making the Diagnosis

Making the diagnosis of prostate cancer takes an alert practitioner, diagnostic studies and ultimately a biopsy. The suspicion of prostate cancer usually comes from the PSA blood test, and/or a digital rectal exam. An ultrasound study is then used to help identify the location of a mass. But only biopsies of the prostate can definitely diagnosis prostate cancer. And this is important to remember. I am going to give only the briefest overview of these tests just so we both understand the conversation we are having. For more information on these tests, as much or as little as you want, please talk to your doctor, check out references in the library or use the various websites online.

THE ULTRASOUND

A Trans rectal ultrasound for the prostate is similar to a vaginal ultrasound that many women have to check their ovaries and uterus. The obvious difference is that with a Trans rectal ultrasound, as the name suggests, the probe is inserted into the man's rectum to check his prostate. As I said before, the rectal ultrasound cannot make or confirm or rule out the diagnosis of prostate cancer. This ultrasound can provide information about the size and shape of the prostate gland and is helpful in directing biopsies to areas of suspicion (hisandherhealth.com). Although uncomfortable there are usually no "after" effects. Sometimes men will have a biopsy at this point. However, if certain medications are taken, such as aspirin, the biopsy will be rescheduled for a later time.

THE BIOPSY

Very simply stated, a biopsy is a procedure that removes tissue or cells for examination under a microscope. A prostate biopsy is a procedure in which samples of prostate gland tissue are removed with a special biopsy needle to determine if cancer or other abnormal cells are present. A biopsy of the prostate is usually done after other diagnostic tests (PSA, digital rectal exam and Trans rectal ultrasound), indicate a problem with the prostate gland. The biopsy is used to confirm the diagnosis of prostate cancer, yet due to the size of the prostate gland, it is possible that a biopsy may reveal "inconclusive" results. This means that in some cases, a diagnosis of cancer cannot be confirmed and it cannot be ruled out. In this situation, very careful surveillance by means of lab studies, rectal exams and possible annual biopsies are performed.

The biopsy procedure is usually performed by an urologist who may use one of three methods (Tran rectal, perineal or transurethral), to obtain tissue samples. Regardless of the method used, the biopsy is usually done on an outpatient basis. The actual method or procedure depends upon the physician as well as the condition of the individual man.

How can we, as women, be of help? Well, that depends upon the people involved. My husband preferred to handle this alone. And he wanted to go right back to work after the procedure. Mark scheduled his biopsy between normal business appointments as an outpatient procedure in the urologist's office.

In my mind, Mark had downplayed the significance of the procedure. I wanted to be there but also wanted to respect his need for control. So, I stayed by the phone. We both rationalized that we wouldn't have the results that day anyway. Later, when Mark was telling me about the procedure, I asked him why he wanted to go alone. Mark said that he thought the biopsy would be similar to the ultrasound and that is why he went to work and then on to the procedure alone. He did not realize that taking a biopsy would require the use of a larger device than during the ultrasound and that it would be somewhat painful as he chose not to have any sedation. Looking back, we really were in a fog.

In hindsight, the best thing you can do is get educated. Give yourself some control by understanding what the biopsy may mean for both of you. Hopefully, the biopsy will provide conclusive answers and you will be able to begin to deal with your own individual situation.

A Detour in Our Conversation

I debated with myself whether to share our experience after the biopsy. I am always hesitant because everyone has a unique situation. In our case, you would think two health profession-als would understand a biopsy procedure and the aftermath.

I remember reading about prostate biopsies thinking at the time that I had no idea what I was reading. It just didn't sink in. I was still trying to adjust to the situation we were in—the fact that my best friend may have cancer. So when we were looking at each other after the biopsy, I wondered why no one told us what a biopsy really means to your sex life.

With that said if you think it may help, continue reading and I apologize if I get a little graphic in my description. If you would rather my thoughts not cloud your own reactions or expectations, please skip *"Our Prostate Biopsy"* and I'll join you again in a few paragraphs.

Our Prostate Biopsy

After a biopsy of prostate tissue, a man may have blood in his urine or stool for a few days. What we didn't know was that a man may also have blood in his semen for days or weeks after the biopsy. It sounds simple doesn't it? No big deal, just some minor drops of blood that will eventually clear itself up. Read-ing words in a book, and hearing words in a busy doctor's office did not translate into reality.

In our case, after the biopsies, there were not just some streaks of red or a minor reddish tinge in Mark's urine or semen. His semen was almost dark brown with blood. Initially we jokingly referred to it as "chocolate ejaculate." A very weak attempt at humor but we were thinking this was just a tempo-rary, two or three day problem. And at the time, we didn't know his biopsy results. What we were unaware of, and perhaps better that we didn't know, was that sex was now over as we knew it.

This was why I debated in sharing our experience. Would it have been helpful if we had known or understood the implications of "blood in your semen for days or weeks" at the time we were going through this? If Mark's biopsy was negative, it would not have made a difference because eventually the blood tinged semen would disappear and our love life would return to normal. But a positive biopsy can have a different effect on your lovemaking.

Waiting for the biopsy results was very difficult. Mark and I have a strong faith founded in our separate religions of Judaism and Catholicism. But never was our faith as strong as during this time. If you believe in God, you know He shows up in mysterious ways. In this particular case, God showed up in two fortune cookies at the end of our Chinese dinner. I kid you not. We opened our cookies and each of us had a unique fortune. Mine said, *"God will help you overcome any hardship."* And Mark's said, *"God looks over you especially."* We've never seen a fortune cookie referring to God before and never have since. But when we read those fortunes, we knew the biopsies would be positive.

We got the news several days later—Mark did have a positive biopsy for cancer. To us that meant that in the three weeks until surgery, we were unable to have normal sexual intercourse because of the blood in Mark's semen. We did try a condom just one time. Condoms were never part of our love life before so it was difficult to use one now. But we gave it a try. It was totally depressing for both of us. We were scared. It made us aware of how much we didn't know and how little control we actually had over this visitor named "cancer" in our lives.

After Mark's surgery for prostate removal, he was unable to have an erection. So basically, the last time we made love was before the biopsy. If I had known that was my last time, what would I have done differently? How come I could not put all the pieces together and understand that we may never make love again and by that I mean intercourse. I am sure I read about it along the way. But it was never emphasized. No one looked directly at me and said this was a possibility. So I am saying to you now…making love before a prostate biopsy may be the last time you both share this experience.

THE DIAGNOSIS

Once we knew the biopsies were positive and we were working with a cancer diagnosis our perspectives changed dramatically. Mark had had a suspicion that there was something wrong for the past two years when his PSA was subtly rising. So even though the diagnosis, "Hit me like a ton of bricks," his worst fears were confirmed and now he was able to move forward making decisions and trying to control the situation. Mark said he felt like he didn't have to worry anymore. His job, money, retirement—none of it was an issue. He had life insurance which he felt comfortable would provide for his family after he was gone. For Mark, the worst case scenario, which was death, was not such a bad alternative. He said the best case scenario gave him more worries than before. The best case scenario would allow him to have all of the normal worries of his life plus living with cancer.

The positive biopsy caught me totally unprepared. When Mark was beginning to get concerned with his PSA results I attributed it to male worrying. I listened but with half an ear. Our children are grown and for the past year or so, we could see the future. We could plan the trips from all of those torn newspaper ads and travel magazines. We could dine out on the weekend with friends or just stay home and snuggle. We had time to hug. We had time to listen to each other and time to make dreams reality. So, what was this? Prostate cancer? I felt totally out of control. I was on the outside trying to understand, to catch up, and to comprehend the situation and just couldn't get a grip on it.

Our urologist was the calming influence. He focused on the positive and was extremely optimistic. He said from the beginning that we were going for a cure. There you have it…three different perspectives, three different lives converging on one diagnosis of prostate cancer.

Implications of the diagnosis

In order to fully understand the diagnosis of prostate cancer, you need to understand the term Gleason Scores. If the biopsy has shown a cancer or malignancy, the Gleason grading system may be used to help describe the appearance of the cancerous prostate tissue. Since this crash course is not intended as a medical reference I will provide only the briefest explanation of Gleason scores. Please speak to your doctor for further information. The best explanation in simple terms I have found is from the Phoenix5 website (http://www.phoenix5.org/articles/menuarticles.html) which is a nonprofit website to help men and their companions overcome the effects of prostate cancer. According to that website, the Gleason grading system assigns a grade to each of the two largest areas of cancer in the tissue samples. Grades range from 1 to 5 with 1 being the least aggressive and 5 the most aggressive. The two grades are added together to produce a Gleason score. A score of 2 to 4 is considered low grade, 5 to 7 is intermediate grade and 8 through 10 is considered high grade. The grade of a prostate cancer specimen is very valuable to doctors in helping them to understand how a particular case of prostate cancer can be treated. In general, the time for which a patient is likely to survive following a diagnosis of prostate cancer is related to the Gleason score. The lower the Gleason score, the better the patient is likely to do. (http://www.phoenix5.org/Infolink/GleasonGrading.html)

My husband's Gleason score was 8. First let me say that our urologist never lost his positive attitude. When we learned that Mark's tumor was so aggressive, our doctor kept saying we were going for a cure. We both found that very comforting. It is so very important to trust your doctor. It goes without saying that the physician you choose is professionally competent, but you also need that gut reaction that you can trust this person. We have all had exams by doctors who clearly have had no personal interest in us nor would they ever remember us when we leave their office. That is not what you want when you are facing prostate cancer.

YOUR CHOICE OF SURGEON

Your choice of doctor will determine the outcome of the surgery as well as your quality of life afterwards. For instance, impotence is one possible complication of removing a man's prostate. Dr. Patrick Walsh is credited with "nerve sparing techniques" which have changed the surgical outcomes for many men. In the past, it was commonly accepted that a man would be impotent following a radical prostatectomy. Today, depending upon the age of the man and if he was sexually active before the surgery, he stands a good chance of being sexually active after surgery. There are other factors during surgery that may affect a man's ability to have an erection, such as blood loss and arterial damage, but a surgeon's experience and skill are also factors to investigate.

Believe it or not a bigger complication than impotence is incontinence or the inability to hold your urine. Imagine at any adult age, the implications and impact on your life if you cannot control your bladder. I don't think I need to say more. It is very important that the urologist/surgeon you choose understands how important bladder control is to both of you and that you talk openly and honestly about this issue ***before*** surgery. Again as much detailed information as you want about the surgery is available online or in various books on the subject.

Most importantly it is beneficial to obtain a second opinion regardless of how much you trust and respect your doctor. Have the biopsy slides checked by another lab. Labs are known to make mistakes, attributable to human error or otherwise. You may have to pay for this consultation but it is well worth every penny. In our situation Mark tried to schedule an appointment with a renowned expert in the field and was refused because his biopsies had a score of a Gleason 8. This "expert" restricted his practice to patients with scores of six or less. Can I tell you how this made us feel? Well I could, but I won't. Undeterred we had the biopsy slides sent to Sloan Kettering for a second opinion which validated the initial report—malignant tumors for a Gleason score of 8.

During this time of waiting for the surgery date, other diagnostic tests are performed in anticipation of surgery. This is a very difficult time to endure. Bone scans are done to determine the presence of cancer outside of the prostate and a Cystoscopy is performed to check the bladder, prostate and urethra. Every time a test turned out to be normal, Mark and I felt hopeful that we would indeed grow old together…a dream that had been badly shaken by the positive biopsies.

FINDING SUPPORT

It is funny but you need to find support wherever it happens to be. Of course you have each other. But each of you has hidden fears and is trying to be strong for the other person. During those three weeks of waiting for surgery, Mark and I discussed the worst case scenario. I guess that comes from working in an Emergency Department but we felt it was better to be prepared for the worst just in case. We discussed our house, should we move now, could I afford to live there if Mark was gone, was there enough life insurance and could we get more. Would our kids be provided for and on and on.

We found our support through family and friends. Our dear friends, Steve and Anna, dropped everything and drove up to our house when we realized we were facing a cancer diagnosis. Group hugs and a glass of wine go a long way in providing comfort. We live a good distance from each other, yet Steve and Anna kept in touch with cards, emails and gifts and many times a heartfelt message on our answering machine.

Mark especially found comfort from a man he knew from the gym whom I'll call George, although that is not his real name. (Mark was still exercising every morning by 5 a.m.) George also had prostate cancer and was quite candid with Mark. George was the only person Mark met who shared his own experience honestly and openly. That person made the difference for Mark because he realized that despite the surgical outcome, he could live with this disease.

For me, the individuals in our family allowed me to lean and lean and lean. Each person offered a different kind of comfort. My Mother listened and helped me understand that I would indeed get through this. My sister listened to my fears and loved me unconditionally. My oldest son Nick hugged me when I had moments of weakness and just couldn't keep it inside anymore. Honestly if he could bottle those hugs, the world would be a better place. My son Chris was away at college but kept in touch each day and stayed with us after Mark's surgery. I should say that during that time I stopped seeing my sons as little boys but got a glimpse of the men they had become.

So you have all of these people around you, loving and supporting you. Yet you are alone in a sense. You may not be able to concentrate. You may find yourself repeating simple chores, leaving cabinet doors open, forgetting where you were going. Give yourself a break. Be kind to yourself. There is no right way to handle this situation. Remember to talk with your best friend—that man in your life. The support of all the people around you allows you to support each other. And right now, you need each other more than ever.

The Surgical Experience

THE TOTAL SURGICAL EXPERIENCE

Depending upon your doctor, you may find yourself choosing between surgery as an outpatient and surgery as an inpatient. If you choose inpatient, patients are usually admitted the morning of surgery and then remain in the hospital for 24–72 hours following the procedure. Outpatients are admitted to the hospital or surgicenter the morning of surgery and are discharged to home on the same day. Mark chose this option however I would strongly recommend staying in the hospital overnight at the very least. But you'll decide for yourself after your own preoperative teaching. Some things to consider are the practical issues. For instance, Mark had to climb a full flight of stairs to get to the bedroom in our house. How does a man who just had major surgery, holding a foley catheter bag, clutching his lower belly and still heavily sedated with pain medication walk up steps?

I have heard both positives and negatives regarding Preoperative teaching. Part of my criticism is that health professionals need to address their level of teaching to the people sitting in front of them. I have discussed this experience with other women and many felt that the preoperative teaching gave them a comfortable overview of their situation. They didn't want to be overwhelmed with specific information. I, on the other hand, arrived with a list of questions hoping for direct answers. I wasn't convinced that a surgicenter was the best place to have a radical prostatectomy so my questions related to infection rates, procedures for emergencies, the "pool" of anesthesiologists and such. I needed to understand Gleason scores. I had high expectations of learning more about the effects of prostate surgery during our preoperative teaching session. Unfortunately, the nurse was unable to answer most of my questions and I left with more anxiety than before the counseling session. Looking back over my notes from that day, very little information was provided as to a "normal" post-operative course. Information related to incontinence, impotence and other potential complications was non-existent. I think I was most surprised that cancer was never discussed. In fact, the word was not mentioned. I was looking for reassurance...support groups, pamphlets, organizations...a plan of support...and there was none.

The one constant, strong force was Mark's surgeon. He had the experience and knowledge that calmed me and gave me confidence in his abilities. When our surgeon said he was going for a cure, I believed him. And so on the morning of October 21st, we left the house at 6 a.m. for Mark's radical prostatectomy. My Mother and I were the only people in the waiting room during the day of surgery. There was no television, no food, no hot coffee or tea. We sat in companionable silence for hours until our doctor came out and told me the cancer was confined to Mark's prostate. He felt confident we would have a cure. My Mother smiled at me, no words were spoken and then we waited awhile longer until Mark was discharged later that day.

I do suggest that you have someone accompany you to the hospital or outpatient facility. It's funny but the night before Mark's surgery the doorbell rang and it was my Mother. My sister and her family had driven two hours to bring my Mother over so I would not be alone the next day in the waiting room. Imagine that. I thought I would go alone and be fine, but my family knew better. You may think you can handle it and you may be just fine, but you owe it to yourself to have that hug waiting just in case.

Looking back it was clear that our perspective on the surgery and life after surgery was cloudy. We really didn't know what a radical prostatectomy meant. We didn't have a frame of reference. And it is difficult to ask questions about a topic that is unfamiliar. It reminded me of when I was a child and always wondered about dictionaries. To be able to use a dictionary, I had to be able to spell the word. If I could spell the word, I wouldn't need a dictionary!

Sitting here two years later and having lived through the experience I now know what to expect and what to explore. What I have come to realize is that people learn in stages. A cancer diagnosis is frightening. Your world stops. You can't breathe. You can't think. When facing surgery, your first impulse is to just "get the cancer out." Act now, ask questions later. What you don't realize is that people live with cancer all of the time.

But at this point in the journey, you are faced with life and death first BEFORE quality of life. I can remember saying to Mark that I can live without sex. And I meant it. Life without my best friend was unthinkable. Rather have him to hold and hug, plan future trips, and share our children's lives than face life alone. Mark said that single statement was the most influential in his decision to have the surgery...sex was not important—life was.

It's not about sex and it is about life. It is time to review your past and what you want for the future. Knowing it will not be the same yet being grateful for the challenge you have and the opportunity for life. At this point it is important to talk with each other which may be easier said than done. The routine of work and family chores may provide a numbing comfort so you don't have to think...to plan...to act. But, it is important to recognize this and begin to plan for change. Support each other by being flexible, being approachable and being responsive to each other.

THE POST-OP COURSE

The first night after Mark's surgery was a very long night. I was afraid to change positions in bed because I did not want to hurt him. Mark was afraid to change positions in bed because of his foley catheter. (This is a tube inserted into the urinary bladder. The urine drains through this tube into a plastic bag attached to the other end.) His list of complaints was endless that night. He was uncomfortable lying down, uncomfortable sitting up, he was nauseous, he was hot, he was cold, he was hurting. And I was scared. Neither one of us slept much. Eventually it was time to get up and face the day…thank goodness.

Activities such as walking are not limited after surgery. Although Mark preferred to stay in bed, I insisted he walk around and sit in the living room. I am a firm believer in sunshine for improving things. And so the hours passed. We kept diligent records of how much fluid Mark drank, and how much urine we emptied from his catheter. We noted when he took antibiotics and how often he needed pain medication. These little chores kept us focused.

Postoperatively we ran into a few situations I will briefly describe.

- The first is that blood-tinged urine in the catheter bag can be more than tinges. It can be almost "rose" in color. Drinking more fluids usually clears this up. If in any doubt, contact the doctor—you are not bothering them. Your questions and concerns are important and legitimate.

- Constipation is a common problem after a radical prostatectomy. A laxative, such as Phillips Milk of Magnesia, is available over the counter and usually works well. You may want to purchase a laxative and any prescriptions for pain medications or antibiotics ahead of time so you are not overwhelmed with yet another errand during this time. Also it is common to have more blood in the foley catheter bag with a bowel movement.

- A surprise to both of us was the swelling and discoloration of Mark's scrotum. Needless to say we were both upset thinking he had internal bleeding. As it turns out, this swelling is another common problem and usually resolves on its own.

- For the first few days following Mark's surgery he had a slight temperature elevation of 101 degrees Fahrenheit. This can be a normal response following surgery and in Mark's case did not indicate an infection or any complication. Again, call your doctor with ANY concerns.

- If you have opted for the outpatient procedure, pain management is essential in the first few days after surgery. No one gets addicted to pain medications by taking them short-term as prescribed following surgery. Mark was hesitant to take Percocet and so waited until his pain was making him very uncomfortable. It is best to keep pain under control and so taking pain medication early is better than waiting.

- Some people are more comfortable lying in a recliner or on the sofa. The key is to be flexible. The bed may be best one day and a recliner the following day. Most important is to move—walk into the kitchen. Get up to change the television channel.

The days following surgery will vary depending upon the procedure as well as all of the things that make us individuals such as our age, medical history, overall health etc. But there are some things we all will have in common to discuss.

Most men, if not all, will be sent home with a foley catheter. This catheter is inserted through a man's penis into his bladder and is used to drain urine from the bladder. Depending upon the surgeon, the catheter will be left in place 7–21 days.

Handling the catheter at home can be a cumbersome experience but manageable. The important thing is to keep the catheter clean and empty the bag that the urine drains down into often. At night, we put an inexpensive plastic trash can (purchased just for this purpose) on the floor beside our bed. The catheter bag fit nicely inside and removed any fear that it would leak or puncture during the night. A foley catheter can be "capped" so the person can shower which is preferred over taking a bath. The surgical nurse should show you how to cap the catheter for this purpose. And don't worry if the two of you are clumsy when you attempt this at home. At the very worst, there will a splash of urine on the floor and a potentially humorous moment for later memories. I can remember Mark and I standing together in our bathroom trying to attach a leg bag (smaller bag that fits under trousers) for his visit to the doctor. I thought to myself, I'm a nurse. What is wrong with me? Why is this so difficult? Looking back, the foley catheter wasn't difficult. The whole situation was difficult. I was tense. I was tired. I was scared.

After the foley catheter is removed, statistics show that many men, especially during the year following surgery, will have some difficulty controlling their flow of urine. That makes it very important to follow the doctor's instructions to regain control of the bladder muscles. It is also important not to underestimate the impact of surgery on this vital area of nerves, tissue, muscles and blood supply. Surgery rearranges things a bit.

Mark made an effort to use the toilet every hour while he was awake. He practiced starting and stopping his urinary stream. And yes, he did not have full control in the weeks following surgery. This incontinence upset Mark more than anything. It changed his routine. When it was time for him to return to work, Mark refused to wear the products marketed for adult incontinence. Instead he chose a small pad which was sufficient in most cases. We learned a lot together. Such as Mark could not control his urine while walking up a flight of stairs. Or that Kegel exercises were recommended but just weren't practical in the weeks following surgery. As much as Mark wanted and needed to get back to work, it took a lot of courage throughout the day to handle incontinence issues.

The other major issue confronting men after prostatectomy surgery is impotence or lack of an erection. Once again this situation is unique to each man depending upon his age, medications and medical history similar to the incontinence issue.

In our situation, there was something in our relationship that I took for granted as so many of us do in a healthy sexual partnership and that is waking to a man with morning erections! So, we went from healthy playfulness to nothing. There was little time to adjust or adapt. It just was sitting there "like the elephant in the room." I learned people are highly adaptable and we adjusted just like many other couples. I will share more on this subject in the next section.

Approximately three months after surgery, Mark told me his penis was bent. I thought to myself, how can a man joke about this? Haven't we been through enough? But I accompanied him into our bedroom and saw for myself. His penis was indeed bent and was painful. Our urologist diagnosed it as Peyronies, a potential complication of surgery, and said that it should stabilize within the year. If the condition progressed and continued to be painful, further surgery would be required!

Mark knew he was not having more surgery, so he did some research on the topic himself. We learned that spontaneous erections during the night and throughout the day serve a purpose of keeping blood flowing. Mark had a radical prostatectomy in October and did not have any type of erection until January, so there were clots from lack of use and from the surgery itself. Mark started a routine of massage around the areas in his penis that contained the scarred tissue and clots. It was very painful for him but he persisted, encouraged by the noticeable improvement in the straightness of his penis.

If I have a pet peeve anywhere in this experience, it has to do with all of the jokes about Viagra, Levitra and Cialis. My pet peeve is the negative connotation associated with these drugs. We all hear about the 80 year old man taking Viagra to have sex with his 70 year old girlfriend. That may be a bonus for some, but I don't believe it was ever the original intention for these drugs. Following a radical prostatectomy, it is part of the post operative treatment for men to take Viagra every day for three months or longer. The purpose is to keep the blood flowing, prevent Peyronies and help restore the normal function of erections. Our insurance company restricted the number of prescriptions, regardless of phone calls to explain the diagnosis of prostate cancer, post operative therapy and the need for daily medication. To make matters worse, samples from our urologist were basically non-existent or Mark would feel uncomfortable asking for the drug.

Speaking of our urologist, the connection between doctor and patient is an interesting relationship after prostate surgery. Our urologist is a man with a very busy practice. The exam rooms are small, the waiting room large and crowded. It is my opinion that urologists need to make time for patients with a cancer diagnosis; time outside of the exam room, perhaps in a room with chairs to sit down and have an honest discussion with the perception that there is time to listen.

Unless the doctor has actually faced cancer, actually had a prostatectomy, then they are not speaking from personal experience. They can only relate book knowledge, experience from performing surgery and comments that their patients pass on to them.

In that respect, their knowledge of a man's ability to have an erection again after prostate surgery is only as good as patients tell them. And male bravado needs to be set aside. This was not an area Mark was comfortable discussing with anyone except two other men who also had a prostatectomy.

But I will say that there is a connection for men between impotence and work. In Mark's case, work was the one place he had control. The one place he was whole. In a way it was his emotional therapy and lifeline for hope. Mark had boundless energy at work. Nothing bothered him or as he said, "Bullshit bounces off." Cancer gave him emotional strength. Yet in the words of another younger man with prostate cancer he felt his coworkers would lose confidence in him if they knew he was now impotent.

Life after Surgery

SO HOW IS SEX AFTER PROSTATE SURGERY?

To answer this question is a very delicate matter. Most people think of sex as intercourse but who really knows what constitutes sex for modern America. But regardless of the method of fulfillment, most people relate a male erection with sex. So let's start there since prostate surgery brings the focus directly on erections. At each office visit after surgery, the urologist asked Mark, "How are the erections?" "How's sex?" Initially, Mark was comfortable to say nothing was happening because we had been told that for the first six months not to expect too much. This turned out to be true. Had the office atmosphere been more conducive to speaking...there were things we wanted to know. Such as how do you make love without horniness or desire? Is sex important when facing a diagnosis of cancer? Obviously life is more important. But as the days and months go by, it becomes very clear that intimacy is a vital part of a marriage. And for us, as for many, sex is part of that intimacy. A man's loss becomes a loss to you as well.

Which brings me to the subject: What does an erection mean to a man? An erection is a natural, normal occurrence most men experience from the time they can remember until well into older age. Most men take erections for granted. They don't think about sexual arousal and erections anymore than they think about breathing. Of course, disease, medications, desire and other factors affect everyone differently.

Now erections and impotence are daily concerns. It is the brain versus the body. According to Laken (2002) desire begins in the brain. The brain sends a signal to the body telling it to respond in the form of an erection. Men take this reaction as a sign of arousal and sexual interest. A prostatectomy damages this physical response leaving the man in uncharted territory. When a man loses his ability to get an erection he loses more than physical functioning. He also loses a part of his emotional and mental self.

The word "impotence" that we heard before surgery became a reality after surgery with even greater significance than we ever considered. A crash course on impotence from our experience involves the following:

- One issue is the fear of intimacy. Regardless of the longevity of your relationship, a man can become afraid. Afraid that he can't live up to expectations and afraid of your rejection. A woman also becomes afraid because she is not sure she is sending the right signals. There is doubt if her man stills finds her attractive...or if he is associating her with cancer....or if he needs someone new to start again and many other worries. A woman is also afraid of initiating sexual behavior for fear of rejection. Imagine after years in a relationship suddenly finding it difficult to hug and lie together. The solution for us was to speak to each other about our sex life, about erections, about our feelings.

- Along with intimacy is the problem of maintaining that couple connection that sex often brings. It is several weeks after successful surgery and life is returning to normal. The daily routine returns except for your sex life. Professional journals and other references recommend oral sex. Have you ever tried oral sex without getting any response from your partner—no erection? The doctors say that it is possible to have an orgasm with a flaccid or limp penis. That may be, but just like a man living with erections his whole life—I was only familiar with an erection as a sign of sexual arousal.

- Our urologist said the vagina is the best stimulation for recovery. What can I say other than we tried to have intercourse only once with a soft penis. It was beyond description.

- These experiences made us realize we needed to try something different or we would lose our sex life forever. We have met other couples who never had sex again after prostate surgery because they did not feel it was worth the effort. This brings me to the very important point that every couple needs to search for their own answers/solutions. It is not something you as a woman can do alone. To discover your own answers/solutions you need to re-educate yourself and your partner. Your man definitely needs to be willing to learn how to do things differently. Because his prostate was removed, his desire was removed. He will need to pay more attention to what his brain is saying and train himself to act on instinct rather than the old ways that don't work anymore. This is easier said than done. The key is not to remember what was…but how it works now. You also need to be patient and learn new ways. In the heat of desire, it is difficult not to interpret a limp penis as rejection.

- Our solution was to turn the focus from sex to "therapy." To protect both of us emotionally and keep us as a team in this recovery, we turned our love life into "therapy." We scheduled regular time each weekend and made it a priority. One example of therapy involved taking showers together to see if Mark could respond to stimulation with any degree of erection. It sounds simple and you probably did this together before prostate surgery but suddenly it takes on a whole new meaning. Removing the "lovemaking" aspect removed the pressure from both of us. Instead we learned together and focused on the physical changes resulting from surgery.

- There are actual physical changes. In our situation, after Mark's surgery his male anatomy seemed "pulled up." His scrotum looked very compact. In Mark's words things felt "less roomy" and "feels like someone else." Initially his testicles were painful and engorged. We later found out that this was from cut seminal vesicles engorged with semen. Another surprise to us was that there was no longer any ejaculate. I'm sure we were told about this somewhere in the process, but it is one thing to be told and another to live with the reality. So now we had a situation of no erection, no ejaculate and no vaginal intercourse.

- In the post-operative period and for months to follow, medications and adjuncts can help with "performance anxiety" and fear of rejection. As previously mentioned, Levitra, Viagra, Cialis and other similar drugs are essential to the recovery of tissue following prostate surgery. As part of Mark's initial post operative visit, he was given a few samples of Viagra as well as a prescription. Mark only used Viagra for a short time before trying Levitra due to the nasal congestion and a feeling of suffocation at night. Levitra was part of Mark's routine for months, with cash payments for the prescription as our insurance company denied the claim. I have to admit that during this time I was very sensitive to the Viagra jokes and even called into a talk show to voice my "knowledge" of prostate cancer and these drugs. Eventually Mark moved on to Cialis and is still using Cialis two years later. We pay approximately $300 for 20 Cialis pills, as our insurance allows us 10 pills for a three month period.

- In addition to these medications, there are various devices or sex toys that may be useful in developing confidence to attempt intercourse. I apologize for the rough language, but we did use "cock rings" with some success. I have to admit that it was the use of these rings that gave us the extra push we needed to attempt intercourse again. After several months and lots of reassurance from me, Mark eventually gave them up. There was a noticeable difference in his erections without the ring but steady improvement each month following surgery.

As I get ready to leave this section on sex after surgery, I cannot stress enough that you need to work together for solutions and persevere. Let me give you an example. Mark's surgery was in October. In the January following Mark's one year anniversary, we took a long anticipated trip to London. Maybe it was the change of location, or the fact that Mark was alternating between Levitra and Cialis, or just that we were relaxed but that was the first time we were able to have sexual intercourse since this all began.

ESTABLISH A ROUTINE

The most important thing I can suggest during that first year is to establish a routine for yourselves as a couple. You both need time to gain perspective on your situation and establish a new intimacy between you. For the man, this may mean waiting for signs of an erection. My husband said he did not realize how important an erection was to being a sexual being. If he was "hard" he would think of sex; if he was not hard, all he would think about was getting hard.

And so during that first year we scheduled sex. This sounds silly, but it provided a safety net for us. And it created motivation. Otherwise, days and weeks could go by without either one of us touching the other or initiating lovemaking. Weekends provided an easy routine for scheduled interludes. I do not want to mislead you into thinking everything was fine. It was not. Reality was a lot of work, attitude and commitment.

As the woman, I made sure the weekend "appointments" worked. I had to remind myself of our earlier relationship and how we used to anticipate spending time together. So, I wrote out notes of invitation to join me for a glass of wine or to join

me on the sofa. I am sure you get the idea. I spent time thinking of special clothes to wear, almost as visual triggers, and not
just for myself but for Mark also. I wanted him to feel loved
and desired. To be honest with you, there were times I was
disheartened and felt burdened by the responsibility of these
weekends. But I remembered how much we had invested
already and would sit down and talk with Mark about it. I
needed to know my efforts were making a difference for him
in regaining his balance both sexually and as a man and husband.

WHERE ARE WE ONE YEAR LATER?

One year after having a radical prostatectomy, we are still heal-
ing and learning how to live with cancer.

Physically Mark's recovery has been smooth. He does not
worry about losing control over his bladder but it is not the
same as before his surgery as every once and awhile…oops!
His incision is 99% healed only because it is located at the
band of his underwear. Overall, the year has gone better than
anticipated.

Our weekends continue to be important. We are still exper-
imenting with our sex life, varying activities trying to take the
focus from erections to lovemaking. I have learned that erections are not tied to Mark's desire for me but I continue to
struggle with Mark's satisfaction as there is no ejaculation of
semen any longer. Oh the things we take for granted.

We did learn that physical intimacy is underestimated and
taken for granted in relationships. Without sex, you can lose

that closeness that intimacy brings and grow apart. During the stress of surgery and the aftermath, you may believe you do not need physical lovemaking. Depending upon your relationship this may be true. We know couples that have given up on their sex life after a prostatectomy because it was too much work and we also know couples who try everything from vacuums to injections to have intercourse. It is truly variable, depending on the individuals involved and their life journey.

Probably the most difficult thing this past year has been the repeat PSA blood tests. Due to the aggressive nature of Mark's tumor, he will have these blood tests frequently during the first two years after surgery to detect the return of prostate cancer and then throughout the remainder of his life. It continues to puzzle me that we are relying upon the very same test that was "normal" prior to Mark's prostatectomy to warn us if the cancer has returned. But I keep reading everything I can about prostate cancer and the PSA continues to be one of the strongest predictors of prostate cancer even after a radical prostatectomy. We have had one huge scare when a PSA result came back that was "normal." The lab technician did not understand why Mark was so upset until he explained that his PSA should be undetectable or zero because he had prostate cancer and subsequent prostate removal. The test was repeated and the PSA did come back as undetectable. That one experience brought us right back to the reality of living with cancer. That test was a wake-up call for me because I realized I was not prepared for Mark's cancer to return. And I had to learn to live with my fear that his cancer might return and I would have to handle it.

It turns out that many people living with cancer are afraid of its return and that this fear of a cancer recurrence is a very common reaction. Researchers are just beginning to understand the psychological ramifications of living with cancer. This is especially true for people with prostate cancer because typically it is a slow growing cancer and many times there are no symptoms. And improvements in screening technology have resulted in earlier detection and treatment allowing men to live years after receiving the cancer diagnosis. Fear of cancer returning is a substantial burden on men who have had a radical prostatectomy, radiation or other treatment for prostate cancer and one that does not diminish over time.

The best advice I can give you is the advice our urologist gave us. After our post-operative visit, he told us to go and live our lives. And that is exactly what we all need to do. You have to make a decision. You have to decide to take control of this situation by educating yourself and by learning how to live with your fears. Every time your husband/partner has a headache or doesn't feel well, you'll be certain the cancer has returned. In the middle of a movie, or while grocery shopping, or driving a car, you'll start to cry as you think about the uncertainty of your life that you are sharing with this man you love.

But then, there will be this imperceptible moment, when you find you are no longer afraid of your partner dying from prostate cancer as you realize that you have both learned how to live with his cancer. It is a goal worth fighting for and it will happen to you too.

Selected Readings

American Cancer Society, (2004). *Cancer Facts and Figures 2004.* Retrieved from http://www.cancer.org/downloads/STT/CAFF_finalPWSecured.pdf.

Boehmer, U., & Clark, J., (2001). Communication about prostate cancer between men and their wives. *The Journal of Family Practice,* 50, 226-31.

Bokhour, B., Clark, J., Inui, T., Silliman, R., & Talcott, J., (2001). Sexuality after treatment for early prostate cancer: Exploring the meanings of "Erectile Dysfunction". *Journal of General Internal Medicine,* 16, 649-55.

Cancer Facts. (2004). The prostate-specific antigen (PSA) test: Questions and answers. *National Cancer Institute.* Retrieved from http://cis.nci.nih.gov/fact/5_29.htm.

Cancer Reference Information. (2005). Detailed guide: Prostate cancer, can prostate cancer be found early? *American Cancer Society.* Retrieved from http://www.cancer.org/docroot/CRI/content/CRI_2_4_3X_Can_prostate_cancer_be_found_early_36.asp?rnav=cri.

Cancer Reference Information (2006). Detailed guide: Prostate cancer, what are the key statistics about prostate cancer? *American Cancer Society.* Retrieved from http://www.cancer.org/docroot/CRI/content/CRI_2_4_1X_What_are_the_key_statistics_for_prostate_cancer_3 6.asp.

Clark, J., Bokhour, B., Inui, T., Silliman, R., & Talcott, J., (2003). Measuring patients' perceptions of the outcomes of treatment for early prostate cancer. *Medical Care,* 41, 923-36.

Davison, J.B., Gleave, M., Goldenberg, L., Degner, L, Hoffart, D., & Berkowitz, J., (2002). Assessing information and decision preferences of men with prostate cancer and their partners. *Cancer Nursing,* 25, 42-49.

Freedland, S., Mangold, L., Walsh, P., & Partin, A., (2005). The prostatic specific antigen era is alive and well: Prostatic specific antigen and biochemical progression following radical prostatectomy. *The Journal of Urology,* 174, 1276-81.

Laken, V & K., (2002). *Making Love Again.* Sandwich, Masschusetts: Ant Hill Press.

Maliski, S., Heilemann, M., & McCorkie, R., (2002). From "Death Sentence" to "Good Cancer": Couples' transformation of a prostate cancer diagnosis. *Nursing Research,* 51, 391-7.

Mehta, S., Lubeck, D., Pasta, D., & Litwin, M., (2003). Fear of cancer recurrence in patients undergoing definitive treatment for prostate cancer: Results from CaPSURE. *The Journal of Urology,* 170, 1931-33.

Thompson, I., Pauler, K., Goodman, P., Tangen, C., Lucia, M.S., Parnes, H.L., Minasian, L.M., et.al., (2004). Prevalence of prostate cancer among men with a prostate-specific antigen level <4.0 ng per milliliter. *New England Journal of Medicine,* 350, 2239-46.

Walsh, P., Worthington, J.F., (2001). *Dr. Patrick Walsh's Guide to Surviving Prostate Cancer.* New York: Warner Books, Inc.

978-0-595-39823-2
0-595-39823-5